M000250716

Alkaline Ketogenic Salads

Over 50 Ridiculously Easy, Nutrient-Packed, Super Healthy & Tasty Recipes You Can Make in 15 Minutes or Less

By Elena Garcia
Copyright Elena Garcia © 2019

Sign up for new books, fresh tips, super healthy recipes, and our latest wellness releases:

www.YourWellnessBooks.com

All rights reserved. No part of this publication may be reproduced, stored in a retrieval system, or transmitted, in any form or by any means, electronic, mechanical, photocopying, recording or otherwise, without the prior written permission of the author and the publishers.

The scanning, uploading, and distribution of this book via the Internet or via any other means without the permission of the author are illegal and punishable by law. Please purchase only authorized electronic editions, and do not participate in or encourage electronic piracy of copyrighted materials.

Disclaimer

A physician has not written the information in this book. It is advisable that you visit a qualified dietician so that you can obtain a highly personalized treatment for your case, especially if you want to lose weight effectively. This book is for informational and educational purposes only and is not intended for medical purposes. Please consult your physician before making any drastic changes to your diet.

All information in this book has been carefully researched and checked for factual accuracy. However, the author and publishers make no warranty, expressed or implied, that the information contained herein is appropriate for every individual, situation or purpose, and assume no responsibility for errors or omission. The reader assumes the risk, and full responsibility for all actions and the author will not be held liable for any loss or damage, whether consequential, incidental, and special or otherwise, that may result from the information presented in this publication.

The book is not intended to provide medical advice or to take the place of medical advice and treatment from your personal physician. Readers are advised to consult their own doctors or other qualified health professionals regarding the treatment of medical conditions. The author shall not be held liable or responsible for any misunderstanding or misuse of the information contained in this book. The information is not intended to diagnose, treat, or cure any disease.

If you suffer from any medical condition, are pregnant, lactating, or on medication, be sure to talk to your doctor before making any drastic changes in your diet and lifestyle.

Contents

Introduction

Thank You for purchasing this book.
It means you are very serious about your health and wellbeing.

Whether your goal is to lose weight, enjoy more energy, or learn a few delicious healing recipes- you have come to the right place.

Alkaline Ketogenic Salads are the easiest and the most effective recipes you can learn to live a healthy lifestyle.

The best part? You don't need any fancy equipment like food processors, blenders or juicers. You can easily make a tasty and nutritious alkaline keto salad in less than 15 minutes.

Heck, many recipes from this book can be even made in 5 minutes, but I didn't want to make such a claim on the title of this book, since some recipes may take a bit longer. Like 7 or 10 minutes!

If you have any experience with cooking or any healthy meal prep, and you already have systems in place to cook at home, you may even discover you can make some of our recipes in less than 5 minutes. Seriously!

Isn't that exciting? Many people think that healthy living and healthy cooking require a ton of time, but it doesn't have to be that way. All you need is your commitment and a simple to follow recipe guide like this one!

So now, let's have a look at alkaline-keto combo...
You are probably thinking...

What?
Alkaline- Ketogenic Mix?
What kind of diet is that?
Can I do it?
Is it easy to follow?
What do the recipes look like?
Are they tasty?

Don't worry. Even if you are a total beginner, and never heard of the keto or alkaline diets, this book will guide you in the right direction.

It's because it is designed for busy people, like you and many others. People who are looking for something simple and effective to follow. This guide (like all of my books) focuses on the HOW so that you can start experiencing positive results of your transformation as soon as possible.

This book is the 4th book in the *Alkaline Keto book series.*

What makes my work incredibly rewarding and fulfilling is reader emails…I love it when my readers share with me how much weight they have lost, or how everyone around them keeps asking them what they have been doing.

Some readers have tried keto diets before, but what they have found much more effective was the alkaline keto combo. Just like some of my readers already tried the hardcore alkaline vegan diet and it didn't work for them in the long run.

What they found effective was incorporating a few of "keto elements" into their alkaline diets and creating a real lifestyle transformation through an alkaline keto combo like described in my Alkaline Keto book series. BALANCE is key!

I originally created the first guide in the series (Alkaline Ketogenic Mix) for my family and friends, because everyone was curious about my own transformation and what I was eating. After realizing how much success my family and friends had with this "hybrid" diet, I knew I could not keep this guide to myself. I wanted to turn it into an easily accessible and affordable program you can jump in and experience all the fantastic health and wellness benefits yourself. And so, this is how the Alkaline Keto book series was born, including Alkaline Ketogenic Mix, Alkaline Ketogenic Salads, Alkaline Ketogenic Juicing, and this book – Alkaline Ketogenic Salads.

Here is precisely what you can expect:

- First, I will introduce you to all the benefits of the alkaline – ketogenic hybrid diet. That will help you get and stay motivated to take massive-inspired action.
- Then, we will dive into an elementary science and practice behind both diets, so that you understand the basics and know what to do without feeling overwhelmed.
- We will also go through certain precautions and common beginner mistakes to avoid. I don't want you to waste your time.

Proper preparation is critical.

-To be successful with this diet, you need to know what to eat, what to avoid, and what you can enjoy in moderation. In this part, you will get very detailed food lists. You will be very positively surprised by how many delicious foods you can enjoy on this diet.

And don't worry! You will not feel hungry or deprived (not at all).

-Finally, you will get a ton of super healthy salad recipes that fuse the best of alkaline and ketogenic diets.

This book is not like a strict program, it's more of a flexible guide, where you can choose your favorite recipes and combine them the way you want. The reason being- if there is a recipe you don't like, and you would need to stick to it, you would lose your motivation. The approach I want to take is freedom and flexibility, while still enjoying, your strong alkaline ketogenic foundation.

So, feel free to pick and choose and enjoy your favorite salad recipes, not only for lunch and dinner but also for breakfast or as a quick, nourishing snack.

Some recipes can also be used as a template to create your own. It may take some time, so at first, you will find the tips helpful. After you have gotten the hang of it, you will know the right food combinations. Then, you will be able to come up with your own recipes, even with your eyes closed.

Ready to transform? Let's do this. I am so excited you are here! Whatever stage you're at, you are in the right place. If you are just starting out, this guide will be a great "shortcut."

And yes, you too can transform with the alkaline keto diet without feeling deprived. Rule number one is -no more restrictive dieting.

No more calorie counting. Eat as much as you want. Eat clean, nourishing food that automatically will help you get rid of sugar cravings and boost your metabolism.

If you are not new to this way of eating, it will inspire you even more and help you optimize your efforts.

After experiencing results and transformation yourself, share this guide with your family and friends to help them too. Everyone deserves to know this information.

Let's start off with keto...what exactly is it? Is the ketogenic diet some new fad?

While the keto diet is definitely more popular these days, it's not a fad. In fact, it's been around for thousands of years, and this is how our ancestors would eat- combining animal products and good fats with some vegetables and herbs.

This is precisely what we will be doing through this guide! We will be embracing the best of the alkaline diet (a ton of fresh nutrient-packed veggies and other healing plant-based foods) with the best of the ketogenic diet (good fats, healthy animal products, and lean protein).

The ketogenic diet has been used clinically since early 1900 to help people with epilepsy.
So what exactly is it?

The simplest definition is:
The ketogenic diet is a diet low in carbs and high in healthy fats.
It encourages to massively reduce the carbohydrate intake and replace it with good, healthy fats (more on healthy vs. unhealthy fats later). This cutback in carbs puts your body into a metabolic state called ketosis.

When in ketosis, your body becomes super-efficient at burning fat for energy. A ketogenic diet can also help reduce blood sugar and insulin levels.

The fact is that we are designed to have periods where we "fast from carbs" and when our glucose levels are depleted.

Then, we start using our body very cleverly, using ketones for fuel. Ketones are the result of our body burning fat for food. The liver converts body fats and ingested fats into ketones.

Transition your diet into a more keto-friendly diet, it's straightforward. It means fewer sugars and carbs and more good fats while eating well!

Following this simple rule (even without going keto full-time) will help you transform your health. It will also help you lose weight naturally if you stay committed to it.

You will no longer be hooked on all those "crappy carbs," and with the new "keto energy," you will feel much more motivated to work out and be more active.

The problem is that in this day and age, we eat way too many carbs and sugars. To make it even worse, we eat processed carbs and sugars (pasta, candy, cakes, etc.). Most people find it hard to start their day without carbs and sugar.

Luckily, once you get into the ketogenic lifestyle, your body is using fat for fuel. The first few days may be a bit weird, but it's like anything, if you give up smoking, drinking...you will feel weird because you are getting rid of toxins. But, looking at the long-term benefits, a ketogenic friendly lifestyle really makes sense as it:
-manages your sugar levels, prevents diabetes
-normalizes your hormones and auto-immune system
-is great for neurological health
-has even been used in clinical settings to prevent Alzheimer's, epilepsies, type 3 diabetes

Also, your brain will thrive. While it can use both glucose and fats for fuel, ketones are a really clean energy source. I can now concentrate much better and for much longer, while feeling less tired because I have transitioned my diet in a more ketogenic friendly direction.
I can now enjoy much more mental clarity; there is no brain fog.

Here are other benefits of aligning your dietary choices with a ketogenic-friendly way:
-you will experience reduced hunger and reduced cravings
-you will be burning fat and reducing carbs and so normalizing your insulin levels

-you will protect your heart while raising the good cholesterol
-you will enjoy the anti-age benefits, as keto foods promote longevity and vitality (while nobody ever promised us we will live forever, by making a decision to stay healthy, we make sure that the time we are here on earth, we feel good and are vibrant).
In other words- burning crappy carbs for energy is like burning dirty fuel while burning fat is a much cleaner fuel while avoiding brain fog. In fact, your brain thrives on ketones.

So here's what the ketogenic diet consists of:
-75%- 80% fat (don't worry, it's all good fat and will not make you fat).
-5-15% healthy, clean protein
-5% good, unprocessed carbs (yea, you can still eat some carbs and the carbs we will be focusing on, will be healthy unprocessed no sugar carbs so no worries, there is no starvation involved here).
While it may seem like something hard to follow, especially when you still got that pasta meal on your mind, it will all become effortless after you get into the creamy, fatty, and actually guilt-free ketogenic friendly recipes!

What is the alkaline diet?

"Going green" is the way to describe an alkaline diet and lifestyle because the focus is on green vegetables in general, as they are the most alkaline food you can ingest.
The benefits of the alkaline diet are numerous. Let us name a few:
WEIGHT LOSS
An alkaline diet will assist you in losing weight. One way that it does this is obvious. The foods you will be eating are very healthy, rich in minerals, and low calorie in general.

Another benefit of an alkaline lifestyle regarding weight loss is that alkaline systems have more oxygen in their cells. Oxygen is a very essential part of eliminating fat cells from the body. The more oxygen in your system, the more efficient your metabolism will be.

ENERGY

Going green does not only give you energy for the apparent reason that you are eating many more healthy, energizing vitamins. You are negating the acid-induced lethargy that is brought on by an unhealthy acid-forming diet.

Not only do our bodies need an abundance of oxygen to lose weight, but we also need oxygen in our cells to energize us. The lack of oxygen in our cells causes fatigue. No, it is not just because you worked too late or partied to hard the night before. It is internal. If your cells are trying to function in a highly acidic environment, they will not be able to transfer oxygen efficiently; leading of course to exhaustion.

Cells in the body also make something that is called adenosine triphosphate (ATP). If your system is very acidic, it harms the ability of your cells to produce it. In the scientific world, it is known as the "energy currency of life." The ATP molecule contains the energy that we need to accomplish most things that we do (both internally and externally).

BODILY FUNCTIONS

Another benefit of the alkaline lifestyle is that your body will be able to function at an optimum level instead of being inhibited by acids:

- Your heartbeat is thrown off by acidic wastes in the body. The stomach suffers greatly from over-acidity.

- The liver's job is to get rid of acid toxins, but also to produce alkaline enzymes. By simply reducing your acid intake, you can internally boost your alkalinity thanks to your liver!
- Your pancreas thrives on alkalinity. Too much acid in your system throws off your pancreas. If you eat alkaline foods, your pancreas can regulate your blood sugars.
- Your kidneys also help to keep your body alkaline. When they are overwhelmed by an acidic diet, they cannot do their job
- The lymph fluids function most efficiently in an alkaline system. They remove acid waste. Acidic systems not only have a slower lymph flow causing acids to be stored; they can also cause acids to be reabsorbed through lymphatic ducts in your intestines that would typically be excreted.

MENTAL FOCUS

The alkalinity of the system is one of the best ways to focus and strengthen the mind. Just as the rest of the body is poorly affected by acid-forming foods and other toxins, so is your brain. And as we all know, it should be possible to control your emotions and decision making with your mind. Guess what? If your body is too acidic and is not alkaline, your mental clarity will be cloudy, your decision making could be off, as well as your emotional state.

DETOX

Another huge benefit of an alkaline lifestyle is detoxification. First, you are going to be cutting out processed foods that are continually adding toxins to your system.

Secondly, you are going to be eating foods that allow your body to detox and rid itself of the acids that have built up in your system all this time. When we detoxify our bodies, our emotions, bodily functions, and mental functions can operate at their optimum levels.

Our bodies function optimally when our blood is at about 7.35 -7.45 pH.
pH levels range from 0 to 14. 0 is the highest level of acidity, but basically, everything 0-7 would be considered acidic. The 7-14 range is alkaline.

Before we dive into complicated pH discussions, here is one thing to understand:
-The alkaline diet is not about changing or "raising" your pH. This is where many alkaline guides go wrong. You see, our body is smart enough to **self-regulate** our pH for us, no matter what we eat.

Unfortunately, when you constantly bombard your body with acid-forming foods (for example, processed foods, fast food, alcohol, sugar, and even too much meat), you torture your body with incredible stress. Why? Well, because it has to work harder to maintain that optimal pH...

Here's a simple example...

Imagine you immerse yourself in a bath filled with ice. You say, but hey, my body can self-regulate its optimal temperature, right? And yes, it can. But it will eventually collapse, and you will get ill. The same happens with nutrition and our blood pH.

You can spend years indulging in toxic, processed, acid-forming foods that only deprive your body of its vital nutrients, saying: "But hey, my body will self-regulate its optimal blood pH."

And again, it will...but sooner or later, it will give up and manifest a disease. It will accumulate fat as its natural defense function to protect your body from over-acidity. We don't wanna end up there, right?

Changing your diet to one that is full of alkaline foods is one of the easiest and best things you can do for your overall health. One of the easiest and most effective ways to do so is with salads. The good news is that you can say goodbye to boring, unappetizing, strictly alkaline salads make of broccoli, tomatoes, and cucumber. We will be eating delicious and filling alkaline keto salads to get you closer to your health goals starting today!

When it comes to the alkaline diet, there is something called the 70/30 rule meaning that about 70% of your diet should be fresh, nutrient-dense alkaline-forming foods and the remaining 30% can be acid-forming foods (however they still should be clean and organic, for example, grass-fed meat or organic eggs).

This is what we will be doing in this book. Or...imagine, some fresh salmon, served with a large avocado, lime juice, and spices. Or...an amazing veggie salad with some naughty bacon and organic cheese.

The basic rule to shift your meals towards an alkaline-keto friendly style is to:
-add more greens to your diet (can be done through salads, or you can juice the greens, or add them to your smoothies).
-add more good fats (for example organic cheese, fish, avocado, coconut oil)

Now, let's have a break from the theory and have a look at the keto food lists. Then, we will have a closer look at the alkaline foods and their role in this lifestyle. The goal is to help you have more energy, enjoy better vitality, and feel fabulous.

Your alkaline-keto-friendly food lists

The following foods can be eaten to your heart's content!
Oh, and when it comes to eating meat, you can choose fattier cuts
with skin and on the bone. In fact, you totally should!

When choosing fish, choose all wild-caught fish with fins and scales.
Industrial fish are full of toxins and not good for you.
All kinds of veggies are excellent, and making sure you serve your
keto meals on heaps of greens will help you stay fully nourished and
prevent sugar cravings too.

Also, please note that the food lists below are designed for an
average, busy person who simply wishes to stay healthy, energized,
or lose some weight. So, they are a bit simplified. If you have any
specific goals, whether it's athletic or healing, any particular health
issue, I would recommend you invest in a dietician specializing in
ketogenic diets and alkaline foods so that they can create
personalized food lists for you and your desired outcome.

Keto - Meat (try to go for organic)
• Beef
• Lamb
• Turkey
• Duck
• Chicken
• Goat
• Venison
• Veal
• Buffalo
• Elk

• As well as **all organ meats such as liver, kidney, etc.** of the above animals

Meat leftovers are a fantastic addition to your green, alkaline-rich salads!

Keto - Fish (try to go for freshly caught)

- Salmon
- Mackerel
- tuna
- haddock
- halibut
- bass
- trout
- sole
- herring
- snapper
- sardines
- whitefish
- whiting

+ as well as a roe from any of these fish
+ Dried and cured meats from the above-mentioned animals and fish are allowed (great for quick salads as well!)

Keto - Eggs and Dairy Products

- organic free-range chicken eggs
- duck and goose organic free-range eggs
- raw full-fat cheeses
- raw cream
- all types of kefir - Raw or organic
- pasteurized cow's milk, goat's milk

- sheep's milk
- *Please note- Dairy products can be skipped if you are lactose intolerant. However, the good news is that if you like cheese, you can use healthy, organic options and add it to your green, vegetable, alkaline-rich salads.*

It's really up to you. Personally, I like to have a little bit of organic cheese or organic kefir every now and then. But, most of the time, I live a dairy-free lifestyle.

Alkaline Keto Veggies
- **All green leafy vegetables:**
- Spinach
- Kale
- swiss chard
- chicory
- romaine and iceberg lettuce
- little gem
- radicchio
- dandelion
- lettuce
- greens,
- chives
- lettuce
- bok choy
- mustard greens
- turnip greens
- nasturtium
- watercress,
- rocket/arugula
- Micro-greens seed sprouts

- Bell pepper

All cruciferous vegetables:
- broccoli
- cabbage
- radish
- kohlrabi
- horseradish
- daikon
- collard greens
- cauliflower
- brussels sprouts
- spring greens

Other non-starchy vegetables:
- artichoke
- asparagus
- avocado
- celery
- endive
- fennel
- garlic
- garlic

Herbs
- Basil
- Cilantro
- Mint
- parsley

Other:

- kelp
- leeks
- okra
- olives
- onion
- spring/green onions
- water
- shallots
- mushrooms (not considered alkaline by most alkaline experts, however, can be added in small amounts and are still keto-friendly).
- chestnuts

Alkaline Grasses

- wheatgrass juice
- barley grass juice

Healthy Keto Fats & Oils (the ones coming from plants are also alkaline)

- Extra-virgin coconut oil
- Extra virgin olive oil (not for cooking)
- Raw butter or ghee
- Grass-fed pasteurized butter or ghee
- Beef tallow
- Goat's milk butter (not for cooking)
- Coconut milk cream (organic, with no additives)
- Coconut butter

Condiments

- All kinds of organic spices, herbs, and pepper
- Unrefined sea salt, Himalaya salt, and rock salt

- Organic Mustard (with no artificial additives)
- Organic Apple cider vinegar
- Balsamic vinegar (with no artificial additives)
- Organic Mayonnaise (made with only natural oils, no vegetable oil)
- Fresh home-made guacamole

Healthy oils and condiments, as well as healing herbs and spices, will not only help you make your alkaline keto salads super healthy, but they will also help you optimize your nutrition.

You can say goodbye to processed, unhealthy, carb, and sugar-loaded condiments that can turn even the healthiest salads into a not-so-healthy meal.

Now, back to our food lists...

If you like pickles, you will be in heaven! You see, an alkaline diet can be very restrictive. For example, fermented foods like pickles and olives are off. This is why I like combining alkaline with keto. The alkaline keto diet is easier to stick to, more enjoyable, tastes delicious, and doesn't make you feel bored.

It's also common sense- it's all about balance, right?

Keto-Friendly Fermented Foods
Pickled vegetables and olives (must be raw, Lacto-fermented)

To be successful with the alkaline keto lifestyle, it's essential to optimize what you drink. You could be eating the healthiest and the most nourishing alkaline keto meals ever...but...if you neglect what you drink and go for processed, sugar, and carb-loaded drinks, you will be spoiling your efforts and hard work.

So, as an extra tip, to help you improve your health and, if desired, start losing weight on the alkaline keto lifestyle (and feel amazing), I highly recommend going for quality hydration, such as:

Drinks
- Filtered water
- Alkaline water
- Herbal infusions (caffeine-free)
- Sparkling mineral water
- Bone broth
- Filtered water with fresh lemon or lime
- Green juice with no high sugar fruit in it (for example celery juice, kale juice, wheatgrass juice)

+ quality tea and coffee is fine in moderation (this diet will help you enjoy more energy naturally, and you don't want to stress your adrenals with an excess of caffeine; coffee as a treat is totally fine though!).

Low Sugar Alkaline & Keto Fruit:
- limes
- lemons
- grapefruits
- pomegranates
- blueberries

Alkaline keto fruit is the healthiest fruit ever because it's low in sugar. It also tastes great in salads or salad salsas. So, don't fear fruit; just go for alkaline keto fruit!

Fats & Oils
- Flax oil (not for cooking)
- Avocado oil (not for cooking)
- Hemp seed oil (not for cooking)
- Walnut oil (not for cooking)
- Expeller-pressed sesame oil (not for cooking)

The healthy, alkaline-keto fats make fabulous and original salad dressings.

Nuts & Seeds

- Flaxseed (raw, ground)
- Sesame seeds
- Tahini (sesame butter)
- Almonds (raw, soaked/sprouted)
- Almond butter
- Brazils (raw, soaked/sprouted)
- Hazelnuts (raw, soaked/sprouted)
- Pecans (raw, soaked/sprouted)
- Pistachio Nuts (raw, soaked/sprouted)
- Walnuts (raw, soaked/sprouted)
- Macadamias (raw, soaked/sprouted)
- Macadamia butter
- Pine Nuts
- Pili nuts
- Chia seeds (raw and soaked)

Nuts are great if you want to reduce your intake of animal products and experiment with a plant-based version of alkaline keto lifestyle. They are also rich in healthy, natural fats and proteins, so feel free to use them as snacks. Ever since I got into nuts, I no longer crave bread!

Have you noticed how the "eat freely" food lists combine organic animal products, good fats and super healthy, chlorophyll-rich alkaline-forming veggies? That's the salad recipe success! You can now combine the pleasure of eating "normal food" with the healing properties of herbs and vegetables. It will no longer feel like a diet, or an ever-lasting cleanse or detox!

The goal of alkaline keto salads is to help your body get back in balance naturally.

No more starvation. And no more stress. You can live a healthy lifestyle and really enjoy it while inspiring those around you! After focusing on what is right for you, and what makes you feel amazing and energized, while restoring balance, it will be automatically so much easier for you to let go of, or reduce the foods and drinks that do not help you achieve your health goals...

Foods to AVOID as much as possible:

Sugars, Sweeteners & Other

- White and brown sugar
- Coconut sugar
- Chocolate
- Raw honey
- Date syrup
- Pure maple syrup
- Molasses
- Tropical fruits
- Fruit juice
- Candy

Drinks

- Alcohol
- Caffeine
- A note about caffeine: 1 quality expresso a day is fine if you really need it. If you do, be sure to stay hydrated throughout the day.

Other foods and drinks to avoid:

All commercial, refined, heat-treated, denatured or artificial foods such as:

- bread
- baked goods
- sauces
- pastries,
- tinned foods
- microwave meals
- fast food
- breakfast cereals

- confectionery,
- sweets
- soy
- processed milk

Other:

All artificial sweeteners:

- Aspartame
- Sucralose
- acesulfame K
- saccharin
- xylitol
- sorbitol
- erythritol
- high-fructose corn syrup
- glucose
- fructose
- Golden syrup
- Agave syrup
- Rice malt syrup

Fats & Oils

All industrial seed oils such as:

- vegetable oil
- canola oil
- cottonseed oil
- rapeseed oil
- corn oil
- sunflower oil
- hydrogenated oil
- safflower oil

- soybean oil
- peanut oil
- Non-extra virgin olive oils
- margarine and spreads
- Lard
- Shortening

Drinks

• All soda drinks, energy drinks, and diet sodas
• Commercial fruit juices and smoothies (even raw)
• Fruit cordials
• Milkshakes and flavored milk
• Artificial alcoholic beverages
• Soya milk

Fruits

• All fruit that is high in sugar

Grains

All grains, gluten, and flours:

- Wheat
- corn,
- rice
- spelt
- rye
- buckwheat
- barley
- oats
- bulgur

Other foods to avoid:
•beans
• lentils
• Peanuts
• Grain-fed meat and dairy
• All grains
• Soy
• Potatoes

Fats to avoid:
-industrial seed oil, trans-fatty acid
- industrial vegetable oil they are very processed, very corrosive to our arteries, they produce heart disease
-Soybean oil
-Sunflower oil
-Cottonseed oil
-Corn oil
-Canola oil (rapeseed oil)

Condiments like mayonnaise also contain the above-mentioned toxic oils, and so do industrially made bakes and goods.
The fast-food industry uses those oils too.

The most common mistakes with the ketogenic diet:
The most common mistake that people make is that they do not include enough veggies with their keto foods. That can cause imbalance and acidity. Hence, I am such a big fan of keto and alkaline diets combined together. Green vegetables are a fantastic addition to your keto diet.

They will help you have more energy and also add more variety to your diet.

The real keto lifestyle is about variety, abundance, and energy. It's hard to be successful with a keto diet if a menu consists entirely of animal products.

The role of alkaline foods
It's essential to get a ton of greens and alkaline foods as these foods are rich in minerals and vitamins while at the same time don't contain sugar.

I have been promoting alkaline foods for years.
They oxygenate your body and help you have more energy and can be combined with other diets such as paleo or keto diet.

In its optimal design, alkaline diet advocates using good plant-based oils such as avocado and olive oil and coconut oil, and it also excludes wheat products and crappy carbs.

Foods that are rich in sugar are also excluded. The alkaline diet includes low sugar fruits (limes, lemons, grapefruits, etc.)

One of the main principles of the alkaline diet is adding a ton of green veggies into your diet. And this book will show you how to do it with delicious and nutritious alkaline keto salads.

Before we dive into the recipes, we would like to offer you free access to our VIP Wellness Newsletter

www.yourwellnessbooks.com/email-newsletter

Here's what you will be receiving:
-healthy, clean food recipes and tips delivered to your email
-motivation and inspiration to help you stay on track
-discounts and giveaways
-notifications about our new books
-healthy eating resources to help you on your journey
-I am a real human, not some big corporation- and so you can answer my emails and ask me questions. I am here to serve You and other Readers!

No Fluff, no spam. Only good and easy to follow info!

Sign up link (copy this link to your phone, or PC):

www.yourwellnessbooks.com/email-newsletter

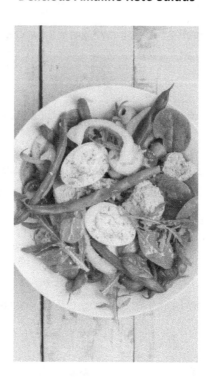

About the Recipes-Measurements Used in the Recipes

The cup measurement I use is the American Cup measurement.
I also use it for dry ingredients. If you are new to it, let me help you:
If you don't have American Cup measures, just use a metric or
imperial liquid measuring jug and fill your jug with your ingredient
to the corresponding level. Here's how to go about it:
1 American Cup= 250ml= 8 Fl.oz.

For example:
If a recipe calls for 1 cup of almonds, simply place your almonds into
your measuring jug until it reaches the 250 ml/8oz marks.
I hope you found it helpful. I know that different countries use
different measurements, and I wanted to make things simple for
you. I have also noticed that very often, those who are used to
American Cup measurements complain about metric sizes and vice
versa. However, if you apply what I have just explained, you will
find it easy to use both.

Recipe #1 Filling Tomato Salmon Salad

Spinach and greens offer iron and chlorophyll, while fresh grapefruits provide a ton of Vitamin C.

Tomatoes offer a variety of alkaline nutrients such as vitamin E, thiamin, niacin, vitamin B6, folate, magnesium, phosphorus, and copper. They're also a source of dietary fiber, vitamin A, vitamin C, vitamin K, potassium, and manganese to help you stay hydrated and energized.

Serves: 2
Ingredients:
For the Salad:
- 4 large carrots, peeled and sliced (or spiralized)
- 4 large tomatoes, sliced
- 1 grapefruit, peeled and chopped
- 1 medium garlic clove, chopped
- A handful of fresh basil leaves
- A handful of fresh baby spinach leaves
- A handful of arugula leaves
- A handful of fresh parsley
- 4 slices of smoked salmon, cut into smaller pieces

For the Dressing:
- 1 tablespoon of olive oil
- 1 tablespoon avocado oil
- Pinch of chili powder
- Pinch of black pepper
- A pinch of Himalayan salt
- 1 teaspoon fresh oregano

Instructions:

1. Combine all the salad ingredients in a big salad bowl and toss well.

2. Mix all the salad dressing ingredients. You can use a small hand blender, or quickly combine and stir all the ingredients in a small bowl.

3. Pour the dressing over the salad, toss well, serve and enjoy!

Recipe #2 Sexy Celery Turkey Salad

This salad offers a unique flavor, it's perfect for a quick aperitif. Celery and other alkaline vegetables combine very well with turkey.

Serves: 2
Ingredients
For the Salad:
- 1 cup of celery, chopped
- 2 small carrots, sliced
- A handful of fresh coriander
- 1 tablespoon of chives (minced)
- 2 tablespoons raisins
- Half cup shredded turkey

For the Dressing:
- 2 tablespoons coconut cream
- 1 teaspoon curry powder
- Half teaspoon ginger powder
- 1 tablespoon of fresh organic lemon juice
- Himalayan sea salt to taste
- A pinch of black pepper

Instructions:
1. Combine all the salad ingredients in a big salad bowl and toss well.
2. Mix all the salad dressing ingredients. You can use a small hand blender, or quickly combine and stir all the ingredients in a small bowl.
3. Pour the dressing over the salad, toss well, serve and enjoy!

Recipe #3 Celery Root Coconut Bacon Salad

This salad is crunchy and filling! Oh, and it's boyfriend and husband approved!

Serves: 1-2
Ingredients
For the Salad:

- 1 medium green apple (skin optional), diced
- 4 tablespoons of chopped almonds
- A handful of Brazil nuts
- A handful of fresh cilantro
- 1 cup arugula leaves
- 4 slices of fried bacon (I fry it in coconut oil)

For the Dressing:

- 2 tablespoons of olive oil
- 2 tablespoons thick coconut milk
- 1 tablespoon apple cider vinegar
- A pinch of Himalayan salt

Instructions:
1. Begin by frying your bacon.
2. In the meantime, combine all the salad ingredients in a salad bowl.
3. Using a small hand blender, combine all the dressing ingredients. You can also combine them in a small cup or bowl and mix well with a spoon until smooth.
4. Add the fried bacon to your salad (make sure it's not too hot).
4. Pour the salad dressing over the salad.
5. Serve and enjoy!

Recipe #4 Delicious Kale Chicken Salad

In this salad, scallions blend amazingly well with kale and chicken. This salad offers good fats and healthy protein to help you stay full for hours.

Serves: 1-2
Ingredients
For the Salad:
- Half cup of pistachios shelled
- 1 cup of kale, chopped
- 4 scallions, thinly sliced
- 1 avocado, peeled, pitted and sliced
- 1 cup shredded chicken

For the dressing:
- ¼ cup of tahini paste
- ¼ cup of coconut milk
- 1 garlic clove
- Himalayan salt, to taste
- Half a lemon, juiced
- 1 tablespoon miso paste

To Garnish:
- A few cilantro leaves
- A few parsley leaves
- A few mint leaves

Instructions:

1. Combine all the salad ingredients in a big salad bowl and toss well.

2. Mix all the salad dressing ingredients. You can use a small hand blender, or quickly combine and stir all the ingredients in a small bowl.

3. Pour the dressing over the salad and toss well.

4. Sprinkle over a few mint, parsley, and cilantro leaves.

5. Serve and enjoy!

Recipe #5 Bell Pepper Greek Cheese Salad

This salad will allow you to enjoy the taste of traditional Greek salad in a super healthy, alkaline-keto friendly version!

Serves: 2
Ingredients
For the Salad:
- 1 large orange bell pepper (cut into smaller pieces)
- 1 large green bell pepper (cut into smaller pieces)
- 1 red bell pepper cut into chunks
- 1 cup of black and green olives, pitted
- 1 green onion, chopped
- ½ cup of organic walnuts, chopped
- 2 medium cucumbers, peeled and sliced
- Half cup cilantro leaves, washed
- Half cup organic feta cheese (you can also use a plant-based version of feta cheese)

Ingredients for the salad dressing:
- 2 tablespoons of olive oil (extra-virgin)
- 2 tablespoons of avocado oil
- 2 tablespoons of apple cider vinegar or Bragg Aminos
- 1 tablespoon of dried organic oregano
- 2 large garlic cloves, peeled and minced
- Half teaspoon of Himalayan salt
- Half teaspoon fresh black pepper

Instructions:

1. Start off by preparing the salad dressing by mixing all the ingredients for the vinaigrette in a small bowl or glass. Stir well with a fork.

2. Next, place all the vegetables into a salad bowl. Toss well. Add the feta cheese if you wish. Pour the salsa over the salad. Toss lightly to coat the vegetables with the vinaigrette.

3. You can serve the salad now or chill it for a few hours before serving.

Recipe #6 Spicy Ginger Salmon Salad

Ginger is well-known for its anti-inflammatory and healing properties. Cucumbers are highly refreshing and very alkaline-forming. Salmon, avocado, nuts, and healthy oils will help you stay full for hours!

Serves: 2
Ingredients
For the Salad:
- 2 cucumbers, peeled and thinly sliced
- 1 tablespoon of grated ginger
- 1 cup arugula leaves
- 1 big avocado, peeled, pitted and sliced
- A handful of crushed almonds
- 2 slices of smoked salmon, cut into smaller pieces

For the Dressing:
- 1 tablespoon olive oil
- 1 tablespoon avocado oil
- 1 tablespoon fresh lime juice
- Black pepper to taste
- Himalayan salt to taste

To garnish:
- A few orange wedges
- A handful of cilantro leaves

Instructions:

1. Combine all the salad ingredients in a big salad bowl and toss well.

2. Mix all the salad dressing ingredients. You can use a small hand blender, or quickly combine and stir all the ingredients in a small bowl.

3. Pour the dressing over the salad and toss well.

4. Sprinkle over a handful of cilantro leaves and garnish with orange wedges.

5. Serve and enjoy!

Recipe #7 From the Sea Mackerel Salad

Wakame is very rich in magnesium, which is considered a highly alkaline-forming mineral.

If you can't find wakame, you can also use nori (same type of seaweed that is used for sushi). Both taste great in alkaline-keto salads!

Serves: 2
Ingredients
For the Salad:
- 1 whole cucumber, thinly sliced
- Half cup of parsley, chopped
- Half cup radish halved
- 2 tablespoons of wakame seaweed, soaked in water as per instructions on the package
- half cup smoked mackerel

For the Dressing:
- Pinch of Himalayan salt, to taste (optional since usually, wakame is already pretty salty)
- 2 tablespoons thick coconut milk
- 2 tablespoons raw coconut vinegar
- 2 garlic cloves, peeled
- 1 tablespoon of olive oil (or grapeseed oil)
- 1 tablespoon lemon juice, freshly squeezed
- Pinch of black pepper, to taste

Instructions:
1. Combine all the salad ingredients in a big salad bowl and toss well.
2. Mix all the salad dressing ingredients using a small blender.
3. Pour the dressing over the salad and stir well.
4. Sprinkle over a few mint, parsley, and cilantro leaves.
5. Serve and enjoy!

Recipe #8 Detox Parsley Salad

Parsley is a miraculous ingredient, full of alkalizing properties. It's full of vitamins K, C, and E as well as iron to help you alkalize and take better care of your skin and eyes. This salad is excellent as a quick detox recipe. But you can always add in some meat or other protein if you wish.

Servings: 1-2
Ingredients
For the Salad:
- 1 cup parsley leaves, chopped
- 4 tablespoons of crushed cashews
- ½ cup cherry tomatoes
- 1 big avocado
- A few onion rings
- A handful of fresh cilantro leaves

For the Dressing:
- 2 tablespoons olive oil
- 2 tablespoons fresh lime juice
- 2 pinches of Himalayan salt
- A handful of fresh basil leaves

Instructions:
1. Combine all the salad ingredients in a big salad bowl and toss well.
2. Blend all the salad dressing ingredients using a small hand blender, make sure the mixture is smooth.
3. Pour the dressing over the salad and toss well.
4. Sprinkle over a few mint, parsley, and cilantro leaves.
5. Serve and enjoy!

Recipe #9 Easy Smoked Chicken Salad

Smoked chicken tastes amazing in crunchy keto salads like this one! If you can't find smoked chicken, you can also use "normal" shredded" chicken or any meat or fish leftovers. This salad recipe is very flexible.

Serves:2
Ingredients
For the Salad:
- 1 can of smoked chicken
- 4 tablespoons of pecans
- ½ cup of grapefruit chunks
- ½ stalk of celery, diced
- 1 avocado, peeled, pitted and sliced

For the Dressing:
- Ground black pepper, to taste
- ½ a lemon, juiced
- Himalayan salt, to taste
- ¼ cup of coconut yogurt
- A few cilantro leaves

Instructions:
1. Combine all the salad ingredients in a big salad bowl and toss well. Set aside.
2.Using a small hand blender, blend all the salad dressing ingredients until smooth.
3. Pour the dressing over the salad and toss well.
5. Serve and enjoy!

Recipe #10 Quick Green Egg Salad

Hard-boiled eggs are quick time savers! They taste great in alkaline-keto salads and will help you stay full longer. Be sure to go for organic, free-range eggs.

Serves: 2
Ingredients:
For the Salad:
• 2 boiled eggs
• ¼ cup of raw walnuts, chopped
• 1 small and ripe avocado (peeled and diced)
• 1 cup mixed leafy greens of your choice

For the Dressing:
- ½ teaspoon of freshly cracked black pepper
- 1 teaspoon of herbs de Provence
- ¼ teaspoon of Himalayan or sea salt
- 2 tablespoons of olive oil
- 2 tablespoons apple cider vinegar
- 2 tablespoons avocado oil

Instructions:
1. Boil the eggs.
2. In the meantime, combine all the salad ingredients in a big salad bowl.
3. Cool down the boiled eggs by putting them in cold water.
4. Now, blend all the dressing ingredients using a small blender.
5. Peel the eggs and add them to the salad. Toss well.
6. Pour the salad dressing over the salad.
7. Toss well, serve and enjoy!

Recipe #11 Arugula Tuna with Lemon Parsley Dressing

This salad offers an incredible mix of clean protein, good fats, and superfood greens. The alkaline keto way!

Serves: 2
Ingredients
For the Salad:

- 1 whole scallion, finely chopped
- 2 cups of fresh arugula, chopped
- 1 avocado, peeled, pitted and sliced
- Fresh chopped parsley for topping
- 2 cans of organic tuna in olive oil

For the dressing:

- 4 tablespoons of thick coconut milk
- 4 tablespoons of parsley, chopped
- 2 tablespoons organic lemon juice
- 2 pinches of Himalayan salt (you can always add more if you need to)
- A pinch of black pepper and chili (optional)
- 1 big garlic clove, peeled

Instructions:
1. Combine all the salad ingredients in a big salad bowl and toss well.
2. Mix all the salad dressing ingredients using a small hand blender,
3. Pour the dressing over the salad and stir well.
5. Serve and enjoy!

Recipe #12 Olive Green Veggie Salad

This salad is an excellent solution if you are looking for a meal replacing salad, something that will keep you full for many hours. It's a great mix of veggies, protein, and healthy, alkaline-keto fats!

Serves: 2
Ingredients
For the Salad:

- A few tablespoons of green olives
- 1 cucumber, peeled and finely chopped
- A few onion rings
- A handful of fresh baby spinach leaves
- 1 big garlic clove, peeled
- Half cup black olives pitted
- A few tomato slices
- A few almonds
- 2 cans of organic tuna

For dressing:
- 2 tablespoons of organic Dijon mustard
- 2 tablespoons of organic olive oil
- A few fresh basil and parsley leaves (optional)
- 1 tablespoon of coconut vinegar
- Black pepper to taste

Instructions:

1. Combine all the salad ingredients in a big salad bowl and toss well.

2. Mix all the salad dressing ingredients. You can use a small hand blender, or quickly combine and stir all the ingredients in a small bowl.

3. Pour the dressing over the salad and toss well.

4. Sprinkle over a few mint, parsley, and cilantro leaves.

5. Serve and enjoy!

Recipe #13 Grilled Chicken Salad with Grapefruit and Avocado

This keto-friendly dish is served with delicious alkaline fruits. It's perfect as a quick, comforting dinner recipe.

Serves:2-3
Ingredients
For the Salad:

- 4 skinless chicken breast halves (remove the bones)
- 8 cups of mixed salad greens
- 1 cup of grapefruit chunks
- 3/4th cup of avocado, peeled and diced
- 3/4th teaspoon of grated fresh ginger

For the Dressing:

- 2 tablespoons of low carb mango chutney
- 2 tablespoons of olive oil
- 2 tablespoons of fresh lime juice
- 1 tablespoon of coconut aminos
- Cooking spray

Instructions:

1. Preheat a grill and grease it with some cooking spray.
2. Take a bowl and combine the coconut aminos, chutney, lime juice, olive oil, and ginger in it. Keep aside.
3. Lay the chicken breast halves on a flat surface and brush those with 2 tablespoons of the chutney mixture.
4. Grill the chicken for 4 minutes on each side while coating lightly with the chutney mixture again on flipping. Remove from grill once done.

5. Cut the chicken into diagonal pieces. Lay the avocado slices, grapefruit, and salad greens on the plate and place the chicken pieces on top to serve. Enjoy!

Recipe #14 Easy Holiday Chicken Salad

This simple salad recipe is great for family occasions or as a quick, comforting dinner.

Serves: 4
Ingredients
For the Salad:
- 4 cups of cooked chicken, cubed
- 1 cup of celery, chopped
- 1 cup of chopped pecans
- 1/2 cup of minced green bell pepper
- 1 1/2 cups of dried cranberries
- 2 fresh green onions, chopped

For the Dressing:
- Half cup of paleo or keto mayonnaise (organic)
- Sea salt, to taste
- 1 teaspoon of paprika
- Ground black pepper, to taste

Instructions:
1. Combine the mayonnaise with seasoning salt and paprika.
2. Add all the veggies and fruits. Then, combine the chicken pieces with the mixture.
3. Insert the salad in the refrigerator and let chill for 1-2 hours before serving.
4. Serve in lettuce leaves cups or in bell pepper cups or over keto-friendly bread.

Recipe #15 Creamy Chicken Salad

This is yet another simple recipe that blends the best out of 2 worlds- alkaline and keto.

Serves: 3-4
Ingredients
For the Salad:

- 3 cups of skinless chicken breasts (no bones), cooked
- 1/3 cup of celery, chopped
- 1/3 cup of paleo unsweetened dried cranberries (organic)
- A handful of smoked almonds
- 6 cups of mixed salad greens
- A pinch of black pepper

For the Dressing:

- 1 tablespoon of lime juice
- 1 tablespoon of Dijon mustard
- 1/2 cup of light paleo-keto mayonnaise
- 1/2 cup Greek-style coconut yogurt
- 1 tablespoon of paleo coconut vinegar
- 1/2 teaspoon of Himalayan salt

Instructions:

1. Mix the mayonnaise with shredded chicken, cranberries, celery, almonds, and the rest.
2. Optional – chill in a fridge.
3. Serve and enjoy!

Recipe #16 Sexy Mediterranean Salmon Salad

This super simple salad is great as a quick lunch or dinner. Cilantro is one of the most alkaline foods ever. But it's very often overlooked. It tastes delicious with salmon, greens, spices, and some keto-allowed mayo! So yummy and tasty!

Serves: 2
Ingredients
For the Salad:
- 4 slices of smoked salmon
- 1 head of butter or romaine lettuce
- 4 tablespoons of fresh cilantro, roughly chopped
- 1 whole red onion, diced
- Sea salt
- Black pepper

For the dressing:
- 2 tablespoons of low carb paleo keto mayonnaise
- 1 whole lemon, juiced
- Sea salt
- Black pepper

Instructions:
1. Combine the salmon with the rest of the ingredients, except the lettuce leaves. Toss well.
2. Serve the salad as it is or chilled in the lettuce "boats."
3. Enjoy!

Recipe #17 Chicken Larb Recipe

Lemongrass is a highly alkalizing herb that will make your dishes taste amazing!

Serves:2
Ingredients
For the Salad:

- 2 cups of ground chicken
- 2 tablespoons of lemongrass (minced or powdered)
- 1/3 cup of mint leaves
- A few chopped cilantro leaves
- 1 cup of green onions, sliced
- 3/4 cup shallots, sliced
- 1 whole head of fresh butter lettuce, cut
- 1 tablespoon of Serrano chili, thinly sliced

For the Dressing:

- 2/3 cup of homemade chicken stock (organic)
- 2/3 cup of fresh lime juice
- 1/3 cup of fish stock (natural)
- 2 teaspoons of low carb chili-garlic sauce
- Himalayan salt, to taste

Instructions:

1. Heat up the chicken stock in a stockpot and drop the ground chicken in it. Simmer the chicken for 6-8 minutes while stirring it occasionally to break the lumps. Add the shallots, lemongrass, green onions, and Serrano chilies.
2. In the meantime, combine the fish sauce, lime juice, and chili garlic sauce in a bowl and set aside (our salad dressing)

3. Stir and cook the chicken for 4-5 minutes or until the shallots turn translucent.
4. Once cooked, drain the entire liquid from the stockpot and then toss the chicken mixture with the chili sauce mixture.
5. Add the rest of the ingredients.
6. Serve and...
7. Enjoy!

Recipe #18 Fat'n' Herbs Alkaline Keto Mix Salad

Another recipe combining meat and veggies in a simple, balanced way!

Serves: 2
Ingredients
For the Salad:
- 4 slices of thick-cut bacon
- 1 whole ripe avocado, peeled pitted and sliced
- 1 cup of asparagus, chopped into 2-3 inch pieces
- Half cup of baby spinach leaves, chopped

For the vinaigrette dressing:
- A few tablespoons of olive oil
- 1 teaspoon Dijon mustard
- 2 tablespoons of paleo balsamic vinegar
- 2 teaspoons rosemary, finely chopped
- 1 large clove garlic (peeled and minced)
- 1 tablespoon of thyme, minced
- 1/2 teaspoon of black pepper
- A pinch of Himalayan salt

Instructions:
1. Cook the bacon over medium heat in a pan until the bacon slices turn brown and crispy. Once that happens, drain the bacon slices from the pan using a slotted spoon and set aside.
2. Chop the asparagus and dump in the same pan over the bacon drippings. Stir fry the asparagus for 4-5 minutes or

until the asparagus gets imbued with the bacon flavors. Turn off the heat once done and set the pan aside.

3. Now dump all the ingredients for the vinaigrette in a small bowl or glass jar and whisk with a metal whisk to get the vinaigrette. The vinaigrette should have a bit emulsified look.

4. Lay the baby spinach leaves over a salad platter and sprinkle the bacon bits over the spinach. Add the avocado slices as well and then drizzle a little bit of vinaigrette on top to serve immediately.

Recipe#19 Easy Avocado Mix Tender Salad

This simple salad is perfect for a healthy breakfast or a guilt-free snack!

Serves:2
Ingredients
For the Salad:
- A handful of crushed almonds
- A handful of crushed cashews
- A handful of blueberries
- 1 whole fresh avocado, peeled, pitted and sliced
- 5 strawberries, sliced

For the Dressing:

- 1 tablespoon coconut oil
- 1 teaspoon cinnamon powder
- Half teaspoon nutmeg
- Half teaspoon vanilla
- 6 tablespoons coconut milk

Instructions:
1. Combine all the salad ingredients in a big salad bowl and toss well.
2. Mix all the salad dressing ingredients using a small hand blender.
3. Pour the dressing over the salad and stir well.
4. Sprinkle over a few mint, parsley, and cilantro leaves.
5. Serve and enjoy!

Recipe #20 Oriental Alkaline Keto Green Salad

This salad is perfect for a quick detox (or alkaline cleanse), or as a side dish!

Serves:2
Ingredients:
Salad:
- 1 cup of fresh spring greens
- 2 handfuls of fresh basil leaves, torn roughly
- 5oz. (150 grams) of fresh cherry tomatoes cut in halves
- 1 whole avocado, peeled, pitted and sliced

For the Dressing:
- 1 tablespoon of olive oil
- A pinch of ground cumin
- 2 tablespoons of fresh lemon juice
- 1 teaspoon curry powder
- A pinch of Himalayan salt
- Half teaspoon of ground coriander

To Garnish:
- A few fresh mint, parsley, and cilantro leaves

Instructions:
1. Combine all the salad ingredients in a big salad bowl and toss well.
2. Mix all the salad dressing ingredients.
3. Pour the dressing over the salad and stir well.
4. Sprinkle over a few mint, parsley, and cilantro leaves. Enjoy!

Recipe #21 Easy Spinach'n' Nuts Salad

This simple plant-based alkaline keto salad is excellent for detox. It can also be served as a simple side dish to help you incorporate more greens into your diet.

Serves:2
Ingredients
For the Salad:
- 2 cups of fresh strawberries, sliced
- 1 cup of fresh baby spinach
- 4 tablespoons of chopped walnuts
- 1 big avocado, peeled, pitted and sliced

Dressing:
- 1 tablespoon of coconut vinegar
- 4 tablespoons of melted coconut oil
- 1/2 teaspoon of paleo Dijon mustard
- Some pepper and Himalayan salt to taste

Instructions:
1. Whisk the coconut oil, Dijon mustard, coconut vinegar, ground black pepper, and sea salt in a bowl until the dressing becomes smooth, and you get a well-combined dressing.
2. Slice the strawberries, chop the walnuts, and slice the avocado.
3. Combine the spinach with walnuts, strawberries, and avocado and drizzle the prepared dressing over the salad.
4. Toss the salad lightly to mix well and serve immediately. Enjoy!

Recipe #22 Roasted Broccoli Creamy Coconut Salad

This salad offers a unique mix of green veggies, creamy dressing, good fats, and healthy protein!

Servings: 2-3
Ingredients
For the Salad:
• 2 cups of broccoli, chopped into florets, cooked or steamed
• ½ cup of green olives
• 2 hard-boiled eggs (cooled down and peeled)
• ½ of an avocado, peeled and sliced
• ½ cup of cherry tomatoes, quartered
• Handful of almonds
• A handful of organic feta cheese, cubed
• Black pepper, to taste

For the Dressing:
• 1 tablespoon of coconut oil
• ½ teaspoon curry powder
• A pinch of sea salt
• 1 tablespoon of organic, keto-friendly mustard
• 1 tablespoon of olive oil

Instructions:
1. Combine all the salad ingredients in a salad bowl. Toss well and set aside.
2. Using a small hand blender, combine all the salad dressing ingredients until smooth.
3. Spread the salad dressing all over the salad, mix well, serve and enjoy!

Recipe #23 Smoked Salmon Green Salad

This salad offers another filling lunch option. Horseradish cream spices it up and gives it a unique flavor.

This salad is perfect as a takeaway lunch that will keep you full until the late afternoon or early evening.

Serves: 2

Ingredients:

- 4 big slices of smoked salmon, cut into smaller pieces
- 1 teaspoon of horseradish cream
- 3 large organic tomatoes, sliced
- 2 small cucumbers, peeled and sliced
- ½ cup of coconut yogurt
- 1 cup fresh watercress
- Juice of 1 lemon
- A dash of ground black pepper
- Himalayan salt to taste

Instructions:

1. Place all the ingredients into a salad bowl. Stir well.
2. Season with black pepper and Himalayan salt to taste.
3. Enjoy!

Recipe #24 Artichoke Alkaline Cleanse Salad

Artichokes are highly alkalizing and full of magnesium and potassium.
They're the perfect ingredient for a healing, refreshing green alkaline salad like this one!

Serves: 1-2
Ingredients:
- 1 cup of canned artichoke hearts, halved
- 1 cup of fresh kale leaves, stemmed and coarsely chopped
- 1 grapefruit, peeled and sliced
- ½ a red onion, sliced
- ½ cup of coconut yogurt
- 2 tablespoons of lime juice
- 2 slices of lime to garnish
- A handful of cashews to garnish
- A handful of cilantro to garnish
- Pinch of Himalayan salt to taste

Instructions:
1. Mix all of the salad ingredients in a large bowl.
2. Stir well while adding the coconut yogurt.
3. Season with Himalayan salt. Garnish with cashews, cilantro, and limes slices. Enjoy!

Recipe #25 Naughty Avocado Dream Salad

This salad is very easy to make, tasty, rich in good fats, and incredibly creamy.

Serves: 1-2
Ingredients
For the Salad:

- Half cup of organic goat cheese
- Half cup crushed cashews
- 1 cup arugula leaves
- 1 whole avocado, peeled, pitted and sliced
- A handful of fresh cilantro

For the Dressing:

- Half cup coconut yogurt or full fat, organic Greek yogurt
- A Pinch of black pepper to taste
- A pinch of sea salt to taste
- 1 lime, juiced

Instructions:
1. Combine all the salad ingredients in a salad bowl. Toss well and set aside.
2.Using a small hand blender, combine all the salad dressing ingredients until smooth.
3. Spread the salad dressing all over the salad, mix well, serve and enjoy!

Recipe #26 Easy Mediterranean Baby Spinach Salad

Spinach is rich in essential minerals and protein as well as high iron content. The vitamin C in the tomatoes helps improve the absorption of iron.

Serves: 1-2
Ingredients:
- 1 cup of raw baby spinach
- 1 cup of raw zucchini, grated
- Half cup of raw cherry tomatoes halved
- A handful of black olives, pitted and halved
- A handful of green olives, pitted and halved

Dressing Ingredients:
- 2 tablespoons of extra virgin olive oil
- Juice of 1 lime
- 2 small garlic cloves
- 1 chili flake
- Pinch of Himalaya salt
- Pinch of black pepper
- 3 segments of orange
- 3 tablespoons thick coconut milk

Instructions:
1. Start off by blending all the dressing ingredients using a blender.
2. Place the raw baby spinach onto a serving plate.
3. Top with the grated zucchini and cherry tomatoes.
4. Add the black and green olives.

5. Pour over the salsa and toss well.
6. Drizzle with the olive oil and serve.

Recipe #27 Cheesy Pumpkin Surprise

The combo of pumpkin and cilantro, along with the pine nuts, and other spices, makes this salad incredibly flavorful.
Organic mozzarella cheese makes this salad taste amazing!

Serves: 2-3
Ingredients:
- Half cup of fresh cilantro, well rinsed and dried with a kitchen towel
- A handful of fresh parsley, well rinsed and dried with a kitchen towel
- 1 cup of pumpkin, cooked, peeled and finely sliced
- Half cup of fresh cherry tomatoes halved
- A few slices of fresh mozzarella cheese, cut into smaller pieces
- Half cup of raw pine nuts

For the Dressing:
- 1 teaspoon of nutmeg powder
- 1 teaspoon of curry powder
- ¼ teaspoon of Himalaya salt to taste
- 1 tablespoon of sesame seed oil

Instructions:
1. Place the fresh cilantro and parsley in a serving bowl.
2. Top with the pumpkin, mozzarella, and cherry tomatoes.
3. Add the raw pine nuts and sprinkle the spices and salt over the top
4. Drizzle with the sesame seed oil and serve.
5. Enjoy!

Recipe #28 Alkaline Green Keto Energy Salad

Turn to this quick, detox salad whenever you need to increase your energy levels! It's fast, natural, tasty, and effective.

Serves: 2-3

Ingredients:
- 1 cup fresh baby spinach leaves
- 1 raw green sweet pepper, sliced
- 1 cup raw cherry tomatoes, halved
- 1 big orange, peeled and segmented
- ¼ cup raw pistachios, roughly chopped
- 1 big ripe avocado, peeled, pitted and sliced
- 2 tablespoons avocado oil

Instructions:
1. Place the baby spinach in a serving bowl.
2. Top with the rest of the ingredients.
3. Add the raw pistachios.
4. Drizzle with the avocado oil, serve.

Recipe #29 Healing Herbs Avocado Salad

The herbs used in this salad make avocado taste amazing, and they also add to the mineral and nutrient content of this salad.

Serves: 2
Ingredients
For the Salad:
- 2 avocados, peeled, halved and pitted
- ¼ cup of mixed Mediterranean herbs (for example thyme, rosemary, basil, oregano, parsley)
- ¼ cup of dried cherry tomatoes, quartered
- ¼ cup of cooked turkey or chicken
- Optional: 1 sheet of nori, cut into smaller pieces

For the Dressing:
- 1 tablespoon of extra virgin avocado oil
- Juice of a half lemon
- Pinch of black pepper and Himalaya salt to taste, if needed

Instructions:
1. Place the avocado halves in a serving bowl.
2. Add the rest of the ingredients.
3. Drizzle with some avocado oil and lemon juice.
4. If needed, season with Himalaya salt and black pepper.
5. Enjoy!

Recipe #30 Easy Spicy Papaya Salad

The combination of spicy chili really compliments the sweetness of the papaya in this recipe. The cashew nuts add a really nice crunch and a hearty dose of protein.

Serves: 1
Ingredients
For the Salad:
- 3 tablespoons of Mediterranean herbs mix
- 1 cup of diced fresh papaya
- 4 fresh cucumbers, finely sliced
- Half teaspoon of fresh red chili powder
- A handful of raw cashew nuts, roughly chopped

For the Dressing:
- 1 tablespoon of virgin olive oil
- A pinch of Himalayan salt

Instructions:
1. Place herbs in a serving bowl.
2. Top with the cucumber, papaya, and cashews.
3. Sprinkle the chopped chili and coconut shavings over the top and toss together.
4. Drizzle with the olive oil and serve.
5. Enjoy!

Recipe #31 Crunchy Alkaline Keto Salad Snack

This salad is another spicy, fruity option with a "multidimensional" taste. The Brazil nuts bring along some crunchy protein. This salad is perfect for a healthy breakfast or a quick snack.

Serves: 2-3
Ingredients:
- Half cup of cilantro, well rinsed and dried off with kitchen towel
- 1 big grapefruit, peeled and cut into smaller pieces
- Half teaspoon of red chili powder
- Half cup of raw Brazil nuts, roughly chopped
- 1 teaspoon of cinnamon powder
- 4 tablespoons of thick coconut milk

Instructions:
1. Place the fresh cilantro leaves into a serving bowl.
2. Top with the pineapple and Brazil nuts.
3. Sprinkle over the chili powder and toss together.
4. Sprinkle over the cinnamon.
5. Drizzle with the coconut milk and serve.
6. Enjoy!

Recipe #32 Arugula Seduction Salad

Here is yet another example of how one can get creative with different flavor combinations while enjoying the healing nutrition of green-alkaline lifestyle.

Serves: 1-2
Ingredients:
- 1 cup of fresh arugula leaves
- 2 avocados, thinly sliced
- A handful of almonds
- Juice of half a lemon
- Half cup raw pecan nuts, roughly chopped
- 1 tablespoon of raw seed mix

Instructions:
1. Place all the ingredients in a salad bowl.
2. Mix well, serve and enjoy!

Recipe #33 Iceberg Hydration Tuna Egg Salad

Lettuce has high water content, and it blends really well with the cucumber. This salad is designed to help you maintain hydration throughout a long hot day while keeping your belly and taste buds satisfied.

Serves: 2-3
Ingredients:
- 1 small iceberg lettuce, washed, dried and chopped
- 4 raw carrots, peeled and thinly sliced, or spiralized
- 4 raw cucumbers, peeled and sliced
- 3 chili flakes, cut into micro pieces (you can also use a half teaspoon of chili powder)
- Half cup of raw pistachios, roughly chopped
- Optional: 2 nori sheets, cut or torn into smaller pieces
- 2 cans of organic tuna
- 2 hard-boiled eggs, cooled down and peeled
- 1 tablespoon of sesame seed oil
- Himalayan salt and black pepper to taste

Instructions:
1. Mix all the ingredients in a big salad bowl.
2. Drizzle with sesame seed oil and, if needed, season with Himalaya salt and black pepper.
3. Enjoy!

Recipe #34 Oriental Creamy Cashew Dream

Fresh iceberg lettuce combines really well with creamy ingredients such as cashews, avocado, and coconut oil. Perfect alkaline keto combo to help you add more healing plant-based foods into your diet.

Serves: 2-3
Ingredients:
- 1 small iceberg lettuce, washed, dried and chopped
- 1 big ripe avocado, peeled, pitted and sliced
- 6 tablespoons of thick coconut milk
- Half cup of raw, unsalted cashew nuts
- 4 tablespoons chopped chives
- Pinch of black pepper, Himalaya salt and chili powder to taste

Instructions:
1. In a medium-sized salad bowl, combine the lettuce, avocado slices, cashews, and chives.
2. Mix well.
3. Now, drizzle with coconut milk and sprinkle some black pepper, Himalaya salt, and chili powder to taste if needed.
4. Toss well, serve and enjoy!

Recipe #35 Green Protein Plant-Based Keto Salad

This salad is pure health. It combines chlorophyll-rich kale that is also a great source of plant-based protein with other natural nutrients and superfood ingredients.

This recipe is just perfect as a takeaway lunch.

Serves: 2
Ingredients:
- 1 cup of fresh kale leaves, washed and chopped, stems removed
- Half cup of raw hazelnuts, roughly chopped
- 3 nori sheets, cut or torn into smaller pieces
- 2 tablespoons of olive oil
- Juice of half lime or lemon
- Optional: Himalaya salt and black pepper to taste
- A few grapefruit or lime wedges, to serve

Instructions:
1. Combine all the ingredients in a medium-sized salad bowl.
2. Sprinkle over some olive oil and fresh lemon or lime juice.
3. Toss well.
4. Serve with a few grapefruit or lime wedges.
5. Enjoy!

Recipe #36 Sweet Pepper Egg Protein Salad

This simple to follow salad recipe proves once again how a healthy, alkaline-keto lifestyle can be both interesting and nutritious.

Serves: 2
Ingredients
For the Salad:
- 1 cup of spinach leaves, washed, dried and chopped
- 1 red sweet pepper, sliced
- 1 yellow sweet pepper, sliced
- 1 orange sweet pepper, sliced
- 1 cup of black olives, pitted and halved
- Half cup of cooked turkey or chicken meat

For the Dressing:
- 2 tablespoons of extra virgin olive oil
- Juice of 1 lemon
- Optional: Himalaya salt to season

Instructions:
1. Place all the salad ingredients in a big salad bowl.
2. Toss well.
3. Drizzle with olive oil and lemon juice.
4. Season with Himalaya salt if needed and toss again.
5. Enjoy!

Recipe #37 Creamy Spinach Blueberry Salad

Coconut milk and avocado, mixed with nutmeg, ginger and cinnamon make this salad incredibly creamy while adding to anti-inflammatory properties and naturally sweet taste.

Serves: 2
Ingredients:
- 1 cup of baby spinach leaves
- 1 cup of fresh blueberries
- Half cup of raw, unsalted cashews

For the Dressing:
- Half of a ripe avocado, peeled and pitted
- Half cup of thick coconut milk
- Half teaspoon of powder
- Half teaspoon of nutmeg powder
- Half teaspoon of ginger powder

Instructions:
1. In a medium-sized salad bowl, combine the spinach, blueberries, and cashews.
2. Mix well.
3. Using a blender, blend avocado, coconut milk, cinnamon, nutmeg, and ginger. Process until smooth.
4. Now, combine the creamy blend with the salad. Enjoy!

Recipe #38 Sexy Red Cabbage Salad

Red cabbage is very high in dietary fiber, making this recipe another energy-sustaining option to keep you going all afternoon.

Serves: 1-2
Ingredients
For the Salad:
- Half cup of raw red cabbage, shredded
- 4 small raw carrots, peeled and grated
- Half cup of red grapes, halved
- Half cup of raw cashews, roughly chopped
- 1 ripe avocado, pitted and sliced

For the Dressing:
- 2 tablespoons of thick cashew or coconut milk
- Fresh juice of 1 lime

Instructions:
1. Place all the ingredients in a medium-sized salad bowl.
2. Drizzle with cashew milk and lime juice.
3. Toss well, serve and enjoy!

Recipe #39 Nori Ratatouille Salad

This recipe is one of my favorite dinner recipes, but it could also be served as lunch. It's jam-packed with vitamins, minerals, and natural protein and super easy to make. Nori tastes great in salad recipes!

Serves: 2
Ingredients
For the Salad:
- 1 cup of fresh cherry tomatoes, halved
- 1 cup of raw, or slightly cooked zucchini, thinly sliced
- 1 small red onion, finely chopped
- 1 clove of fresh garlic, finely chopped
- 2 nori sheets, torn or cut into smaller pieces
- A handful of fresh basil leaves, finely chopped
- 1 cup of black olives, pitted and halved
- A handful of raw pine nuts

For the Dressing:
- 2 tablespoons of extra virgin olive oil
- 2 tablespoons of fresh tomato juice
- Optional: Himalaya salt and black pepper to taste.

Instructions:
1. Place the cherry tomatoes in a serving bowl.
2. Add the chopped onion, garlic, and fresh basil.
3. Add the black olives, nuts, and nori.
4. Drizzle over the olive oil and tomato juice.
5. Toss together. Season with black pepper and Himalaya salt if needed. Enjoy!

Recipe #40 Curry Love Chicken Salad

This salad takes advantage of the anti-inflammatory benefits of curry spice while sneaking in some greens full of alkaline benefits.

Serves: 2-3
Ingredients
For the Salad:
•½ cup cooked chicken meat, cut in smaller pieces
•1 cup radicchio
•A handful of walnut halves
•1 large celery rib, halved lengthwise and thinly sliced crosswise
•¼ cup of mixed baby greens

For the Dressing:
•1 teaspoon of curry powder
•½ teaspoon of black pepper
•Himalayan salt to season
•2 tablespoons of coconut vinegar

Instructions:
1. Place all the ingredients in a large salad bowl and stir well.
2. Season with some Himalayan salt and serve right away or cool down in the fridge for a few hours.
3. Enjoy!

Recipe #41 Fatty Creamy Salmon Full on Keto Salad

Salads are not boring! There is always room for creativity, taste, and "creaminess."

Serves: 1-2
Ingredients
For the Salad:

- ½ cup chopped cooked salmon pieces
- 1 cup of mixed salad greens
- 1 green apple, peeled and sliced
- 1 tablespoon of olive oil or grapeseed oil
- 1 small avocado, peeled and diced

For the Dressing:
- 2 tablespoons of fresh lime juice
- 1 tablespoon of coconut aminos
- 1 teaspoon of grated fresh ginger
- A handful of cashews to garnish
- Pinch of Himalayan salt to taste

Instructions:
1. Place all the ingredients into a salad bowl.
2. Pour over olive or grapeseed oil, lime juice, and coconut aminos.
3. Stir well.
4. Season with Himalayan salt.
5. Sprinkle over some cashews to garnish.
6. Serve fresh and enjoy!

Recipe #42 Cranberry Super Green Egg Salad

Cranberries bring in some unique flavor here and spice the salad up! They are also very rich in antioxidants to help you enjoy a healthier and more energized life.

Serves: 1-2
Ingredients
For the Salad:
- 1 cup of celery, chopped
- 1 cup of chopped pecans
- 2 hard-boiled eggs, peel removed
- ½ cup of minced green bell pepper
- 1 cup of cranberries
- 1 fresh green onion, chopped

For the Dressing:
- 1 teaspoon of paprika
- Ground black pepper, to taste
- 2 tablespoons lemon juice
- 2 tablespoons olive oil
- 4 tablespoons of keto-friendly, organic mayonnaise
- Himalayan salt, to taste

Instructions:
1. Place all the ingredients in a salad bowl.
2. Mix well to ensure all the ingredients are equally seasoned.
3. Serve right away and enjoy or store in the fridge for later.

Recipe #43 Spicy Cilantro Salmon Salad

Not only is cilantro highly alkalizing, but it also brings some unique flavor to this salad!

Serves: 1-2
Ingredients
For the Salad:
• 4 big slices of smoked or cooked salmon, cut into smaller pieces
• A few leaves of romaine lettuce, chopped
• Half a lemon, juiced
• 4 tablespoons of fresh cilantro, roughly chopped
• half of red onion, diced
• 1 small red bell pepper, chopped
• 1 cucumber, peeled and chopped
• 1 clove of garlic
• half of avocado, peeled and sliced

For the Dressing:
• 4 tablespoons of coconut cream
• Pinch of Himalayan salt to taste
• Black pepper to taste

Instructions:
1. Place all the ingredients into a salad bowl, adding lemon juice, coconut cream, Himalayan salt, and black pepper.
2. Serve right away or store in a fridge and serve slightly chilled.
3. Enjoy!

Recipe #44 Vitamin C Alkaline Keto Power Salad (great for breakfast!)

This delicious smoothie is jam-packed with vitamin C coming from alkaline and keto-friendly fruits like limes and lemons. It uses natural herbs such as stevia and cinnamon for natural sweetness. This salad is perfect as a quick energy boost and a real aid for your immune system.

Servings: 2
Ingredients:
- 1 big avocado, peeled, pitted and sliced
- Half lemon, peeled and sliced
- 1 cup of coconut milk
- 1 teaspoon coconut oil
- A few drops of liquid stevia to sweeten
- Pinch of nutmeg powder
- Pinch of cinnamon powder
- Pinch of vanilla powder
- A few slices of lime to garnish

Instructions:
1. Place all the ingredients in a salad bowl.
2. Mix well. If needed, add more stevia to sweeten.
3. Garnish with a few lime slices.
4. Serve and enjoy!

Recipe#45 Green Mineral Total Wellness Salad

This recipe can be used both as a smoothie as well as a soup. Whenever I am pressed for time, I make it for dinner, to enjoy something warm, and keep the raw leftovers to have a nourishing green smoothie in the morning.

Servings: 1-2
Ingredients:
- 1 big cucumber, peeled
- 1 small avocado, peeled and pitted
- A handful of parsley
- A handful of cilantro
- 1 cup of thick coconut milk
- A handful of raw cashews
- 1 tablespoon of olive oil
- Himalayan salt to taste
- 1 chili flake

Instructions:
1. Combine all the ingredients in a salad bowl.

2. Toss well, serve and enjoy!

3. You can also blend it and serve it as a smoothie (smoothies can be quicker than salads).

Recipe#46 White Creamy Alkaline Energy Salad

This simple recipe uses healing alkaline veggies like cauliflower, and, at the same time, adds in some garlic to help you strengthen your immune system.

Servings: 1-2
Ingredients
For the Salad:

- 1 cup cauliflower, slightly cooked or steamed, cut into smaller pieces
- Half cup cilantro leaves
- Half cup cashews
- 4 tablespoons melted organic butter (you can also use coconut oil instead)
- 2 garlic cloves, peeled and minced
- Himalaya salt to taste

Instructions:

1. Combine all the ingredients in a salad bowl.
2. Toss well and make sure the cauliflower is smeared in butter or coconut oil.
3. Place the cilantro and cashews on top.
4. Serve and enjoy!

Recipe #47 Anti-Flu Mediterranean Salad

This simple salad is full of anti-inflammatory properties, and it also helps fight colds and flu.

Servings: 1-2
Ingredients
For the Salad:
- 4 medium-sized tomatoes, peeled
- 1 big garlic clove, peeled
- 4 small celery sticks
- A handful of black olives
- 1 hard-boiled egg (optional)

For the Salad Dressing:
- Himalaya salt to taste
- 1 teaspoon oregano
- A few fresh basil leaves
- 2 tablespoons olive oil

Instructions:
1. Combine all the dressing ingredients in a blender. Set aside.
2. Place all the salad ingredients in a salad bowl.
3. Pour the dressing over the salad, toss well.
4. Serve and enjoy!

Recipe #48 Almost Sushi Alkaline Keto Salad

Nori is an excellent source of Iron as well as Omega 3 Fatty Acids and vitamins A & C., And it tastes so delicious in salads!

Servings: 1-2
Ingredients:
- 4 slices of fresh, smoked salmon
- 1 big avocado, peeled, pitted and sliced
- 2 big nori sheets, cut into smaller pieces
- 2 cucumbers, peeled and sliced
- 2 tablespoons avocado oil
- 2 tablespoons fresh lime or lemon juice
- Himalaya salt to taste

Instructions:
1. Combine all the ingredients in a small salad bowl.
2. Add the Himalaya salt, avocado oil, and some fresh lime (or lemon juice).
3. Serve and enjoy!

Recipe #49 Green Power Plants Salad

This salad can be prepared in 2 different versions- vegetarian or with meat.

Servings: 2-3
Ingredients:
Salad Base:

- 1 cup arugula leaves, washed
- 1 small avocado, peeled, pitted and sliced
- 2 cucumbers, peeled and sliced
- 1 tablespoon fresh lemon juice
- 2 tablespoons olive oil
- Himalaya salt and black pepper to taste

Option 1- Vegetarian
2 hard-boiled eggs (shell removed)
A few (fat) slices of goat cheese
Option 2 – Meat or Fish
Half cup of any meat or fish leftovers you have (chicken, beef, salmon).

Instructions:
1. In a big salad bowl, combine all the ingredients from the "salad base."
2. Sprinkle with lemon juice and olive oil.
3. Add Himalaya salt. Toss well.
4. Now add in the rest of the ingredients of your choice (option 1 or 2, or both if you like).
5. Serve and enjoy!

Recipe #50 Irresistible Vegetarían Mediterranean Salad

This salad is perfect if you are pressed for time and are looking for a quick and healthy way to put a nice, nourishing meal together.

Servings: 2
Ingredients:
- 1 cup of mixed greens
- 2 tomatoes, sliced
- A few onion rings
- 6 big slices of goat cheese (preferably organic)
- A few slices of avocado
- Half cup of green olives
- 1 can of tuna (organic)
- 1 tablespoon lemon juice
- 2 tablespoons olive oil (organic)

Instructions:
1. Mix all the ingredients in a big salad bowl.
2. Sprinkle with olive oil and lemon juice.
3. Toss well, serve and enjoy!

Recipe #51 Easy Creamy Warm Salmon Salad

Salmon is definitely one of my favorite keto ingredients, especially to use for quick, nourishing salads like this one.

Servings: 1-2
Ingredients:
- Half cup raw cashews, crushed
- 4 slices of smoked salmon
- 2 tablespoons of coconut oil or butter
- 1 cup fresh spinach
- 2 tomatoes, sliced
- Himalaya salt and black pepper to taste
- A few thin slices of cheddar cheese

Instructions:
1. Place coconut oil in a frying pan.
2. Switch on the heat (medium heat).
3. Add the spinach and Himalaya salt and stir-fry until soft.
4. Now, add the salmon, cashews, and tomato slices.
5. Stir fry until the salmon is warm.
6. Take off the heat and place in a salad bowl.
7. If needed, add more Himalaya salt to taste.
8. Top up with some cheddar cheese, serve and enjoy!

Recipe #52 Alkaline Keto Protein Salad

Eggs can be a real lifesaver, especially for quick alkaline keto salads that are rich in protein.

I like to boil the eggs in bulk to make sure I always have 1 or 2 to add to my salad.

Servings: 1-2
Ingredients:
- 2 hard-boiled eggs, peeled
- 1 cup of mixed greens of your choice
- A few onion springs
- 1 green bell pepper, sliced
- 1 small avocado, peeled and pitted
- 1 small garlic clove
- 2 tablespoons olive oil
- 2 tablespoons water

Instructions:
1. Combine the eggs and greens in a salad bowl.
2. Add the onion springs.
3. Now, using a small hand blender, blend the avocado, with olive oil, water, and Himalaya salt.
4. Spread the avocado dressing onto the salad, toss well, serve and enjoy!

Recipe #53 Arugula Vitamin C and A Salad

Grapefruit is a fantastic fruit that is both alkaline and keto-friendly. It's because it is full of alkaline minerals like magnesium and potassium, while at the same time, it's a low sugar fruit. Exactly what we want on this diet and lifestyle!

Servings: 1-2
Ingredients:
- Half cup fresh parsley
- 1 grapefruit, peeled
- 1 cup arugula leaves
- Half avocado
- 1 can of organic tuna
- Himalaya salt to taste
- 2 tablespoons of avocado or olive oil

Instructions:
1. Combine all the ingredients in a salad bowl.
2. Toss well, serve and enjoy!

Bonus - Eating Out While on Alkaline Keto Mix Lifestyle

Good news, my Dears!
It's actually very easy...

1. If possible, check the restaurant's menu online before booking. (although this is not always necessary as even most "normal" restaurants will have alkaline keto foods on their list).
2. Go for a big, green salad (perfect as an appetizer) with some fish or meat. Or just a vegetable salad with olive oil. You could also indulge in a little bit of cheese. Another option is – meat or fish with vegetables (no potatoes).
3. Be sure to avoid any processed salad dressings. Instead, ask for a raw salad with some olive oil, spices, and lemon juice.
4. As for drinks, order water with lemon or herbal infusion. Most restaurants do offer herbal teas.
5. Occasional treats like a glass of wine, expresso, or even a little dessert are absolutely fine. Although I would keep treats only for special social occasions.
6. Most restaurants will be pleased to customize their menu and services to your needs, so don't be shy, always ask if they can re-modify some of their meals for you. It's as simple as getting rid of that sugar and carb-filled salad salsa or getting rid of potatoes and artificial seasoning to make your meal more alkaline-keto friendly.
Questions:
You can email me at:
info@yourwellnessbooks.com

We Need Your Help

One more thing, before you go, could you please do us a quick favor?

It would be great if you could leave us a short review on Amazon.

Don't worry, it doesn't have to be long. One sentence is enough.

Let others know your favorite recipes and who you think this book can help.

Your opinion is important.

Thank You for your support!

Join Our VIP Readers' Newsletter to Boost Your Wellbeing
Would you like to be notified about our new health and wellness books?

How about receiving them at deeply discounted prices? And before anyone else?

What about awesome giveaways, latest health tips, and motivation?

If that is something you are interested in, please visit the link below to join our newsletter:

www.yourwellnessbooks.com/email-newsletter

It's 100% free + spam free, and you can easily unsubscribe whenever you want.

We promise we will only email you with valuable and relevant information, delicious recipes, motivational tips, and more!

Sign up link:

www.yourwellnessbooks.com/email-newsletter

More Books by Elena Garcia:
www.YourWellnessBooks.com

More Books & Resources in the Healthy Lifestyle Series
These books are available on Amazon in eBook, paperback and audiobook format.

You will find them by looking for *Elena Garcia* in your local Amazon store, or by Visiting:

www.yourwellnessbooks.com

CPSIA information can be obtained
at www.ICGtesting.com
Printed in the USA
BVHW042105231120
594080BV00007B/51

9 781913 857202